HOW TO LOSE WEIGHT IN A WAY YOU CAN MAINTAIN

The Getting Rid Diet.

Michael Samuel

TABLE OF CONTENTS

INTRODUCTION

1.

WELCOME TO THE GETTING RID DIET

The Philosophy of Sustainable Weight Loss

Welcome to "The Getting Rid Diet," a book that is not just about losing weight, but about transforming your life in a sustainable, healthy way. Our philosophy is simple: focus on getting rid of unhealthy habits, negative mindsets, and unsustainable practices, and replace them with positive, lasting changes. This isn't about quick fixes or extreme restrictions; it's about creating a lifestyle that you can maintain for the long term.

Sustainable weight loss is rooted in understanding your body, making informed food choices, and adopting a balanced approach to nutrition and exercise. It's about making small, manageable changes that add up to significant, lasting results. Throughout this book, you'll learn how to nourish your body, enjoy your meals, and live an active, fulfilling life—all while reaching your weight loss goals.

Why Most Diets Fail

The world is full of diets promising quick and dramatic results, but the reality is that most of them fail. Why? Because they often rely on restrictive eating patterns, unrealistic expectations, and temporary solutions. Many diets encourage you to cut out entire food groups, drastically reduce calorie intake, or follow rigid meal plans that are difficult to maintain.

These approaches can lead to initial weight loss, but they are not sustainable in the long run. Once the diet ends, old habits often resurface, leading to weight regain. Furthermore, extreme diets can harm your metabolism, deplete your energy levels, and negatively impact your mental and emotional well-being.

In contrast, "The Getting Rid Diet" focuses on building a healthy relationship with food and understanding the nutritional needs of your body. It's about finding balance, enjoying a variety of foods, and listening to your body's hunger and fullness cues. By adopting a more flexible and realistic approach, you can achieve lasting weight loss and overall well-being.

The Importance of a Healthy Mindset

A healthy mindset is crucial for successful and sustainable weight loss. It's not just about what you eat or how much you exercise; it's also about how you think and feel about yourself and your journey. Negative self-talk, unrealistic expectations, and a focus on perfection can sabotage your efforts and make it challenging to stay on track.

In "The Getting Rid Diet," we emphasize the importance of cultivating a positive and compassionate mindset. This means setting realistic goals, celebrating small victories, and being kind to yourself when setbacks occur. It's about understanding that progress is not always linear and that every step, no matter how small, is a step in the right direction.

By focusing on your overall well-being rather than just the number on the scale, you can develop a more positive and empowering relationship with food, exercise, and your body. This mindset shift is essential for maintaining your progress and enjoying a healthier, happier life.

In this book, we will guide you through the principles and practices of "The Getting Rid Diet," providing practical tips, scientific insights, and motivational support to help you on your journey. Let's get started on a path to sustainable weight loss and a healthier, more fulfilling life.

PART I:

UNDERSTANDING WEIGHT LOSS

2.

THE SCIENCE OF WEIGHT LOSS

Calories In vs. Calories Out

At its core, weight loss revolves around the fundamental principle of energy balance: calories in vs. calories out. This concept is straightforward—when you consume more calories than your body needs, the excess is stored as fat, leading to weight gain. Conversely, when you consume fewer calories than your body uses, your body taps into stored fat for energy, resulting in weight loss.

Understanding this balance is crucial for effective weight management. It's not just about cutting calories indiscriminately but about finding the right balance that allows you to lose weight while still providing your body with the necessary nutrients and energy to function optimally. Throughout this book, we will explore how to create a healthy calorie deficit that promotes weight loss without compromising your overall health and well-being.

Metabolism and Its Role

Metabolism refers to the chemical processes your body uses to convert food into energy. These processes are crucial for maintaining basic bodily functions, such as breathing, circulating blood, and repairing cells. Your basal metabolic rate (BMR) is the number of calories your body needs to perform these basic functions at rest.

Several factors influence your metabolism, including age, sex, muscle mass, and genetic factors. Generally, muscle tissue burns more calories than fat tissue, even at rest, so increasing your muscle mass can help boost your metabolism. Additionally, certain lifestyle factors, such as regular physical activity and a balanced diet, can also positively impact your metabolic rate.

Understanding how your metabolism works and what influences it can help you make informed decisions about your diet and exercise routines. This knowledge will enable you to optimize your weight loss efforts and achieve your goals more effectively.

The Role of Hormones in Weight Management

Hormones play a significant role in regulating hunger, satiety, and fat storage, all of which are crucial factors in weight management. Key hormones involved in these processes include insulin, leptin, ghrelin, and cortisol.

- Insulin: Produced by the pancreas, insulin helps regulate blood sugar levels. When you eat, insulin levels rise, helping cells absorb glucose for energy. Excess glucose is stored as fat. Insulin resistance, a condition where cells don't respond well to insulin, can lead to weight gain and difficulty losing weight.

- Leptin: Known as the "satiety hormone," leptin is produced by fat cells and signals to your brain when you are full. However, in cases of leptin resistance, which can occur in obese individuals, the brain doesn't receive the signal, leading to overeating and weight gain.

- Ghrelin: Often called the "hunger hormone," ghrelin is produced in the stomach and signals hunger to the brain. Ghrelin levels rise before meals and fall after eating. Managing ghrelin levels through balanced meals and regular eating patterns can help control hunger and support weight loss.

- Cortisol: Known as the "stress hormone," cortisol is released in response to stress. Chronic stress and elevated cortisol levels can lead to increased appetite and cravings for high-calorie foods, contributing to weight gain.

Understanding the role of these hormones and how they interact with your body's weight regulation mechanisms can provide valuable insights into your weight loss journey. By addressing hormonal imbalances through diet, exercise, and stress management, you can create a more favorable environment for sustainable weight loss.

In the following chapters, we will delve deeper into these scientific principles and provide practical strategies for applying them to your weight loss journey. By understanding the science behind weight loss, you can make informed decisions and set yourself up for long-term success.

3.

COMMON MYTHS ABOUT DIETING

Dieting is often surrounded by misinformation and myths that can lead to confusion and frustration. In this chapter, we will debunk some of the most common myths about dieting, clarify the roles of macronutrients like carbohydrates, fats, and proteins, and explore the truth about so-called metabolism boosters.

Debunking Popular Diet Myths

Myth 1: Carbs Are the Enemy

One of the most pervasive myths is that carbohydrates are inherently bad and must be avoided to lose weight. While it's true that some high-sugar, low-nutrient carbs can contribute to weight gain, not all carbs are created equal.

Complex carbohydrates, such as whole grains, vegetables, and legumes, provide essential nutrients, fiber, and sustained energy. The key is to choose nutrient-dense, whole-food sources of carbohydrates and watch portion sizes.

Myth 2: Fat Makes You Fat

The belief that dietary fat directly translates to body fat is another common misconception. Healthy fats, such as those found in avocados, nuts, seeds, and olive oil, are vital for overall health, including brain function, hormone production, and nutrient absorption. It's the type and quality of fat that matters, not just the quantity. Trans fats and excessive saturated fats should be limited, while healthy fats should be included in a balanced diet.

Myth 3: Skipping Meals Helps You Lose Weight

Skipping meals can lead to overeating later in the day, making it counterproductive for weight loss. It can also slow down your metabolism as your body conserves energy in response to perceived food scarcity. Regular, balanced meals help maintain stable blood sugar levels, control hunger, and provide the nutrients your body needs to function optimally.

Myth 4: Eating Late at Night Causes Weight Gain

The idea that eating after a certain time automatically leads to weight gain is a myth. What matters more is the total number of calories consumed throughout the day and the quality of the food. While it's true that people may tend to snack on less healthy options late at night, it's the excess calories and poor food choices that contribute to weight gain, not the timing of the meals.

Understanding Carbs, Fats, and Proteins

Carbohydrates

Carbohydrates are the body's primary source of energy. They can be classified into two main types: simple and complex. Simple carbs, found in sugary foods and refined grains, provide quick energy but can lead to blood sugar spikes. Complex carbs, found in whole grains, vegetables, and legumes, are digested more slowly, providing sustained energy and promoting satiety. Including a balance of complex carbohydrates in your diet is important for long-term health and weight management.

Fats

Fats are essential for many bodily functions, including hormone production, nutrient absorption, and cell structure. There are different types of fats, including saturated, unsaturated, and trans fats. Unsaturated fats, found in olive oil, nuts, seeds, and fatty fish, are beneficial for heart health and should be included in a balanced diet. Saturated fats, found in animal products and some plant oils, should be consumed in moderation. Trans fats, often found in processed foods, should be avoided as they can increase the risk of heart disease.

Proteins

Proteins are crucial for building and repairing tissues, producing enzymes and hormones, and supporting immune function. They are composed of amino acids, some of which the body cannot produce on its own and must be obtained through diet. Protein sources include meat, poultry, fish, dairy, legumes, and plant-based proteins like tofu and quinoa. Including a variety of protein sources in your diet helps ensure you get all the essential amino acids and supports muscle maintenance and growth.

The Truth About Metabolism Boosters

Many products and diets claim to boost metabolism, promising rapid weight loss. However, the reality is more complex. Metabolism boosters like caffeine, green tea, and certain spices can have a modest effect on increasing metabolic rate, but the impact is usually small and temporary. There is no magic pill or food that will significantly speed up your metabolism for sustained weight loss.

The most effective ways to support a healthy metabolism are:

1. Building Lean Muscle Mass: Muscle tissue burns more calories at rest than fat tissue. Engaging in regular strength training exercises can help increase muscle mass and boost your basal metabolic rate.

2. Regular Physical Activity: Incorporating a mix of cardiovascular and strength training exercises can help increase overall calorie expenditure and support a healthy metabolism.

3. Eating Regular Meals: Eating balanced meals and snacks throughout the day can help maintain stable blood sugar levels and prevent metabolic slowdowns.

4. Getting Enough Sleep: Lack of sleep can negatively impact metabolism and increase hunger hormones, leading to overeating.

By understanding these concepts and debunking common myths, you can make more informed decisions about your diet and lifestyle, setting yourself up for successful and sustainable weight loss.

PART II: THE GETTING RID DIET PRINCIPLES
4. THE FOUNDATION: BUILDING HEALTHY HABITS

Part II: The Getting Rid Diet Principles

4. The Foundation: Building Healthy Habits

Building a solid foundation of healthy habits is essential for achieving and maintaining long-term weight loss. The Getting Rid Diet emphasizes sustainable changes that can be maintained throughout your life, rather than quick fixes or extreme measures. In this chapter, we will explore the importance of setting realistic goals, developing a positive relationship with food, and practicing mindful eating.

Setting Realistic Goals

Setting realistic and achievable goals is a crucial first step in any weight loss journey. Unrealistic expectations can lead to disappointment and frustration, making it more likely that you will abandon your efforts. Instead, focus on setting specific, measurable, attainable, relevant, and time-bound (SMART) goals. For example, rather than aiming to lose a large amount of weight in a short period, set a goal to lose a modest amount, such as 1-2 pounds per week, which is considered safe and sustainable.

In addition to weight loss goals, consider setting goals related to other aspects of your health and well-being, such as increasing your physical activity, improving your dietary habits, or reducing stress. Remember that progress is not always linear, and it's important to celebrate small victories along the way.

Developing a Positive Relationship with Food

A positive relationship with food is vital for long-term success. Many people struggle with emotional eating, food guilt, or restrictive eating patterns that can lead to an unhealthy relationship with food. The Getting Rid Diet encourages a balanced and flexible approach to eating, where no food is off-limits and all foods can fit into a healthy diet.

Instead of labeling foods as "good" or "bad," focus on the nutritional value and how they make you feel. Allow yourself to enjoy your favorite foods in moderation without guilt. This balanced approach can help you avoid the cycle of restriction and bingeing that often accompanies traditional diets.

Developing a positive relationship with food also involves understanding your body's hunger and fullness cues. Learning to eat when you're hungry and stop when you're satisfied can help you better manage your intake and avoid overeating.

Mindful Eating: Listening to Your Body

Mindful eating is a practice that encourages you to be present and aware during meals. It involves paying attention to the taste, texture, and aroma of your food, as well as recognizing your body's hunger and fullness signals. Mindful eating can help you develop a more intuitive relationship with food and improve your overall eating experience.

To practice mindful eating, start by eliminating distractions during meals, such as watching TV or scrolling through your phone. Focus on your food and take time to savor each bite. Chew slowly and thoroughly, and pause between bites to assess your hunger level. This practice can help you better recognize when you are full and prevent overeating.

Mindful eating also encourages you to be aware of the emotions and thoughts that may influence your eating habits. For example, you might notice that you tend to reach for comfort foods when you're stressed or bored. By becoming more aware of these patterns, you can find healthier ways to cope with emotions and make more conscious food choices.

In summary, the foundation of the Getting Rid Diet is built on setting realistic goals, developing a positive relationship with food, and practicing mindful eating. By focusing on these principles, you can create a sustainable and enjoyable approach to weight loss that supports your overall health and well-being. In the next chapters, we will delve deeper into creating a personalized plan, managing portion sizes, and developing a balanced eating pattern.

5.

CREATING YOUR PERSONALIZED PLAN

In order to achieve sustainable weight loss and maintain a healthy lifestyle, it's crucial to create a personalized plan that fits your unique needs, preferences, and goals. This plan should consider your current eating habits, the role of macronutrients and micronutrients, and practical strategies for meal planning and preparation. This chapter will guide you through these steps, helping you tailor a plan that works for you.

Assessing Your Current Eating Habits

The first step in creating a personalized plan is to assess your current eating habits. This involves taking an honest look at what, when, and why you eat. Keeping a food diary for a week can be a helpful tool in this process. Record everything you eat and drink, including portion sizes, and note any patterns or triggers that influence your eating behavior, such as stress, boredom, or social situations.

Consider the following questions as you review your food diary:

- 1. What types of foods do you typically eat? Are they mostly processed or whole foods? Do you get enough fruits, vegetables, and whole grains?
- 2. How balanced are your meals? Are you including a good mix of proteins, healthy fats, and carbohydrates?
- 3. What are your eating patterns? Do you eat regular meals, or do you tend to skip meals and snack frequently?
- 4. How do you feel after eating? Do you often feel full, satisfied, or still hungry? Do certain foods make you feel sluggish or energized?

Understanding your current eating habits is essential for identifying areas for improvement and making sustainable changes.

The Role of Macronutrients and Micronutrients

A balanced diet includes a variety of macronutrients and micronutrients, each of which plays a specific role in your body's function and overall health.

Macronutrients

1. Carbohydrates: Carbs are the body's primary source of energy. They should primarily come from complex sources like whole grains, vegetables, and legumes, which provide fiber and essential nutrients.

2. Proteins: Proteins are essential for building and repairing tissues, producing enzymes and hormones, and supporting immune function. Include a variety of protein sources, such as lean

meats, poultry, fish, dairy, legumes, and plant-based proteins like tofu and quinoa.

3. Fats: Fats are vital for hormone production, nutrient absorption, and overall health. Focus on healthy fats from sources like avocados, nuts, seeds, and olive oil. Limit saturated and trans fats, which can increase the risk of heart disease.

Micronutrients

Vitamins and minerals, also known as micronutrients, are essential for numerous bodily functions, including immune support, bone health, and energy production. A varied diet rich in fruits, vegetables, whole grains, lean proteins, and healthy fats will generally provide the necessary micronutrients. In some cases, you may need to consider supplements, but it's best to get these nutrients from food whenever possible.

Meal Planning and Prep Tips

Meal planning and preparation are key components of a successful and sustainable diet. They help you make healthier choices, save time, and avoid the temptation of unhealthy convenience foods. Here are some tips for effective meal planning and prep:

1. Set Aside Time for Planning: Dedicate a specific day each week to plan your meals and snacks. Consider your schedule and any special events that may require adjustments.

2. Create a Balanced Menu: Ensure that each meal includes a good mix of macronutrients. For example, a balanced meal might include lean protein, a complex carbohydrate, healthy fat, and plenty of vegetables.

3. Make a Shopping List: Based on your meal plan, create a shopping list of the ingredients you'll need. Stick to the list to avoid impulse purchases and ensure you have everything you need for the week.

4. Prep Ahead: Prepare meals and snacks in advance to make healthy eating more convenient. You can cook and portion out meals for the week, chop vegetables for easy access, and prepare snacks like fruit or yogurt in advance.

5. Use Batch Cooking: Cooking larger portions of meals and freezing them in individual servings can save time and ensure you always have a healthy option on hand.

6. Stay Flexible: While planning is important, be flexible and willing to adjust your plan as needed. Life can be unpredictable, and it's okay to make changes when necessary.

By assessing your current eating habits, understanding the role of macronutrients and micronutrients, and implementing practical meal planning and prep strategies, you can create a personalized plan that supports your weight loss goals and promotes overall health. The next chapter will focus on portion control and establishing regular eating patterns to further support your journey.

6.

PORTION CONTROL AND EATING PATTERNS

Mastering portion control and establishing regular eating patterns are essential components of a sustainable weight loss plan. They help regulate calorie intake, maintain energy levels, and support overall well-being. In this chapter, we will explore how to understand portion sizes, the benefits of regular meal times, and strategies for handling cravings and emotional eating.

Understanding Portion Sizes

One of the biggest challenges in weight management is accurately estimating portion sizes. Over time, portion sizes have increased, leading to a corresponding increase in calorie intake. Learning to recognize appropriate portion sizes can help you manage your calorie intake without feeling deprived.

Tips for Understanding and Managing Portion Sizes:

1. Use Measuring Tools: Use measuring cups, spoons, and a food scale to familiarize yourself with standard portion sizes. This can help you develop a better sense of appropriate portions over time.

2. Visual Cues: Use common objects as visual references for portion sizes. For example, a serving of meat or poultry should be about the size of a deck of cards, while a serving of rice or pasta should be roughly the size of a tennis ball.

3. Read Nutrition Labels: Pay attention to the serving size on nutrition labels and measure out that amount. Be mindful that packages often contain multiple servings.

4. Portion Control Plates: Consider using plates with portion control sections to help guide your servings of protein, vegetables, and carbohydrates.

5. Mindful Eating: Slow down and savor your food, paying attention to hunger and fullness cues. This can help you avoid overeating and better enjoy your meals.

The Benefits of Regular Meal Times

Eating regular meals and snacks at consistent times throughout the day offers several benefits for weight management and overall health:

1. Stable Blood Sugar Levels: Regular eating patterns help maintain stable blood sugar levels, which can prevent energy crashes and excessive hunger, reducing the likelihood of overeating.

2. Improved Digestion: Eating at consistent times supports your body's natural digestive

rhythms, helping to optimize nutrient absorption and digestive health.

3. Better Appetite Control: Scheduled meals and snacks can help regulate your appetite, making it easier to recognize true hunger and avoid mindless eating.

4. Enhanced Metabolism: Regular meals can support a healthy metabolism by preventing long periods of fasting that might cause your body to conserve energy.

To establish regular eating patterns, aim for three balanced meals and one to two snacks per day. Listen to your body's hunger and fullness signals, and adjust your meal times as needed based on your schedule and activity level.

How to Handle Cravings and Emotional Eating

Cravings and emotional eating can be significant challenges on a weight loss journey. It's important to recognize the difference between physical hunger and emotional hunger, and to develop strategies for managing these triggers.

Managing Cravings:

1. Identify Triggers: Pay attention to the situations, emotions, or environments that trigger your cravings. This awareness can help you address the underlying causes.

2. Healthy Alternatives: Keep healthy snacks on hand, such as fruits, vegetables, nuts, or yogurt, to satisfy cravings without derailing your progress.

3. Stay Hydrated: Sometimes, thirst can be mistaken for hunger. Drink water throughout the day to stay hydrated and help curb cravings.

4. Allow for Moderation: It's okay to indulge in your favorite treats occasionally. The key is moderation and mindful enjoyment without guilt.

Managing Emotional Eating:

1. Recognize Emotional Hunger: Emotional hunger often comes on suddenly and is accompanied by specific cravings, while physical hunger builds gradually and can be satisfied with a variety of foods.

2. Find Alternative Coping Mechanisms: Instead of turning to food for comfort, find healthier ways to cope with emotions, such as exercising, meditating, journaling, or talking to a friend.

3. Practice Mindful Eating: Before reaching for food, take a moment to assess whether you're truly hungry or eating out of emotion. Mindful eating can help you make more conscious food choices.

4. Seek Support: If emotional eating is a frequent challenge, consider seeking support from a therapist or counselor who can help you develop healthier coping strategies.

By understanding portion sizes, establishing regular meal times, and learning to manage cravings and emotional eating, you can create a balanced and sustainable approach to eating. These strategies will support your weight loss goals and help you develop a healthier relationship with food. In the next chapter, we will explore the role of exercise and physical activity in weight management and overall well-being.

PART III:

PRACTICAL STRATEGIES FOR WEIGHT LOSS

7.

Exercise and Physical Activity

Physical activity is a crucial component of a healthy lifestyle and an effective tool for weight loss. Regular exercise not only helps burn calories but also improves overall health, boosts mood, and enhances quality of life. This chapter will guide you in finding the right type of exercise for you, explore the benefits of both strength training and cardiovascular exercises, and offer tips for incorporating more physical activity into your daily routine.

Finding the Right Exercise for You

Choosing an exercise routine that you enjoy is key to maintaining consistency and achieving long-term success. The best exercise is one that fits your interests, lifestyle, and fitness level. Consider the following factors when selecting your exercise regimen:

1. Interests and Enjoyment: Choose activities that you find fun and engaging. This could be anything from dancing and hiking to swimming and cycling. Enjoyable activities are more likely to become a regular part of your routine.

2. Fitness Level: Start with exercises that match your current fitness level. As you progress, you can gradually increase the intensity and duration. If you're new to exercise, consider starting with low-impact activities like walking or yoga.

3. Schedule and Accessibility: Select activities that fit your schedule and are easily accessible. If you have limited time, consider short,

high-intensity workouts or exercises you can do at home.

4. Variety: Incorporate a variety of exercises to keep things interesting and work different muscle groups. This can also help prevent burnout and reduce the risk of injury.

The Benefits of Strength Training and Cardio

A well-rounded exercise program includes both strength training and cardiovascular (cardio) exercises, each offering unique benefits for weight loss and overall health.

Strength Training

1. Increased Muscle Mass: Strength training helps build and maintain muscle mass, which is metabolically active tissue. More muscle mass means you burn more calories at rest, which can aid in weight loss.

2. Improved Bone Density: Weight-bearing exercises, such as lifting weights, can increase bone density and reduce the risk of osteoporosis.

3. Enhanced Metabolic Health: Strength training can improve insulin sensitivity, blood sugar control, and cholesterol levels, contributing to overall metabolic health.

4. Functional Fitness: Building strength enhances your ability to perform everyday activities, reducing the risk of injury and improving quality of life.

Cardiovascular Exercise

1. Calorie Burn: Cardio exercises, such as running, cycling, and swimming, are effective for burning calories and supporting weight loss.

2. Heart Health: Regular cardio exercise strengthens the heart and improves cardiovascular health, reducing the risk of heart disease.

3. Endurance and Stamina: Cardio workouts improve endurance and stamina, allowing you to perform physical activities for longer periods without fatigue.

4. Mood and Mental Health: Cardio exercise releases endorphins, which can help reduce stress, anxiety, and depression.

For optimal results, aim for a balanced mix of strength training and cardio exercises. For example, you might do strength training two to three times a week and cardio on the remaining days.

Incorporating Physical Activity into Your Daily Routine

In addition to structured workouts, incorporating more physical activity into your daily routine can help increase your overall energy expenditure and support weight loss. Here are some practical tips:

1. Take the Stairs: Opt for stairs instead of elevators or escalators whenever possible.

2. Walk or Bike: Walk or bike to nearby destinations instead of driving. If you commute, consider getting off the bus or train a stop early and walking the rest of the way.

3. Active Breaks: Take short breaks throughout the day to stretch, walk, or do light exercises. This is especially important if you have a sedentary job.

4. Household Chores: Engage in household chores like cleaning, gardening, or washing the car, which can be a good source of physical activity.

5. Active Socializing: Instead of meeting friends for coffee or a meal, consider active outings like hiking, bowling, or playing a sport.

6. Use Technology: Utilize fitness trackers or apps to monitor your activity levels and set goals. These tools can motivate you to move more throughout the day.

By finding exercises you enjoy, incorporating a balance of strength training and cardio, and increasing your daily physical activity, you can create a comprehensive fitness plan that supports your weight loss goals and enhances your overall health. The next chapter will discuss the importance of sleep, stress management, and hydration in your weight loss journey.

8.

MANAGING STRESS AND SLEEP

Stress and sleep play a significant role in your overall health and weight management. Chronic stress and poor sleep can impact your body's ability to regulate appetite, metabolism, and overall well-being. This chapter will explore the connection between stress, sleep, and weight, offer techniques for reducing stress, and emphasize the importance of quality sleep.

The Connection Between Stress, Sleep, and Weight

Stress and Weight

Chronic stress can lead to weight gain or difficulty losing weight through several mechanisms:

1. Increased Appetite: Stress triggers the release of cortisol, a hormone that can increase appetite and cravings for high-calorie, sugary foods.
2. Emotional Eating: Many people turn to food for comfort during stressful times, leading to overeating and poor food choices.
3. Metabolic Changes: Prolonged stress can lead to metabolic changes that promote fat storage, especially around the abdominal area.

Sleep and Weight

Quality sleep is essential for maintaining a healthy weight and overall health:

1. Hormone Regulation: Poor sleep can disrupt the balance of hunger hormones such as ghrelin (which stimulates appetite) and leptin (which signals fullness). This imbalance can lead to increased hunger and overeating.
2. Metabolic Rate: Inadequate sleep can lower your resting metabolic rate, making it harder to burn calories efficiently.

3. Insulin Sensitivity: Poor sleep can impair insulin sensitivity, increasing the risk of weight gain and type 2 diabetes.

Techniques for Reducing Stress

Managing stress effectively can improve your overall health and support weight management. Consider the following techniques:

1. Exercise Regularly: Physical activity is a powerful stress reliever. Aim for activities you enjoy, such as walking, swimming, or yoga, to help reduce stress levels.

2. Practice Mindfulness and Meditation: Mindfulness practices, such as meditation, deep breathing exercises, and progressive muscle relaxation, can help calm your mind and reduce stress.

3. Stay Organized: Stress often comes from feeling overwhelmed. Use tools like planners,

to-do lists, and time management techniques to stay organized and reduce stress.

4. Connect with Others: Social support is crucial for managing stress. Spend time with friends and family, or consider joining a support group or community organization.

5. Pursue Hobbies: Engage in activities that you find relaxing and enjoyable, such as reading, painting, or gardening. Hobbies can provide a mental break and help reduce stress.

6. Set Boundaries: Learn to say no and set boundaries to avoid overcommitting yourself. Prioritize self-care and make time for relaxation.

The Importance of Quality Sleep

Quality sleep is essential for weight management and overall health. Consider these strategies to improve your sleep:

1. Establish a Consistent Sleep Schedule: Go to bed and wake up at the same time every day, even on weekends, to regulate your body's internal clock.

2. Create a Relaxing Bedtime Routine: Develop a calming pre-sleep routine, such as reading a book, taking a warm bath, or practicing relaxation techniques, to signal to your body that it's time to wind down.

3. Optimize Your Sleep Environment: Ensure your bedroom is conducive to sleep by keeping it cool, dark, and quiet. Invest in a comfortable mattress and pillows.

4. Limit Screen Time: Reduce exposure to screens (phones, computers, TVs) at least an hour before bedtime, as the blue light emitted can interfere with melatonin production and disrupt sleep.

5. Avoid Stimulants: Limit the intake of caffeine and nicotine, especially in the afternoon and

evening, as they can interfere with your ability to fall asleep.

6. Watch Your Diet: Avoid large meals and heavy, spicy foods close to bedtime, as they can cause discomfort and disrupt sleep.

7. Manage Stress: Addressing stress and anxiety through the techniques mentioned earlier can also improve sleep quality.

By understanding the connection between stress, sleep, and weight, and implementing strategies to manage stress and improve sleep, you can enhance your overall well-being and support your weight loss goals. The next chapter will cover strategies for staying motivated and overcoming obstacles in your weight loss journey.

9.

SOCIAL SITUATIONS AND EATING OUT

Social events and dining out can present challenges to maintaining healthy eating habits, but with the right strategies, you can stay on track with your weight loss goals. This chapter provides guidance on navigating social situations and holidays, making healthy choices at restaurants, and employing strategies to stay committed to your goals.

Navigating Social Events and Holidays

Social gatherings and holidays often involve tempting foods and festive celebrations that can derail your weight loss efforts. Here are some strategies to help you enjoy these events while staying on track:

1. Plan Ahead: If you know you'll be attending a social event, plan your meals and snacks for the day to accommodate the special occasion. You might eat a lighter meal before the event to avoid arriving overly hungry.

2. Choose Wisely: At social events, survey the food options before filling your plate. Opt for healthier choices like vegetables, lean proteins, and whole grains. Enjoy smaller portions of richer, higher-calorie foods.

3. Practice Mindful Eating: Focus on the social aspects of the event rather than solely on the food. Eat slowly and savor each bite, paying attention to your hunger and fullness cues.

4. Bring a Healthy Dish: Offer to bring a healthy dish to the event. This ensures you have at least one nutritious option and can introduce others to healthier alternatives.

5. Set Boundaries: It's okay to politely decline offers of additional food or drinks if you're not

hungry. Setting boundaries helps you stay in control without feeling deprived.

Making Healthy Choices at Restaurants

Eating out can be challenging, but with a few smart strategies, you can make healthier choices at restaurants:

1. Review the Menu: Check the restaurant's menu online before you go to identify healthier options. Look for dishes that are grilled, baked, or steamed rather than fried or creamy.

2. Ask for Modifications: Don't hesitate to ask for modifications to make dishes healthier. For example, request dressings and sauces on the side, substitute vegetables for fries, or ask for smaller portions.

3. Watch Portion Sizes: Restaurant portions are often larger than standard servings. Consider sharing a dish, ordering a smaller portion, or

asking for a to-go box and saving half of your meal for later.

4. Choose Balanced Meals: Aim to include a good mix of protein, vegetables, and whole grains in your meal. Avoid dishes that are overly processed or high in saturated fats and sugars.

5. Be Mindful of Beverages: Be cautious with sugary drinks and alcohol. Opt for water, unsweetened beverages, or a small glass of wine if desired.

Strategies for Staying on Track

Maintaining your weight loss goals in the face of social situations and dining out requires planning and flexibility. Consider these strategies to stay committed:

1. Set Realistic Goals: Understand that it's okay to enjoy occasional indulgences. The key is moderation and balance. Set realistic

expectations for yourself and focus on making healthier choices most of the time.

2. Stay Active: Incorporate physical activity into your routine, even if it's just a short walk after a meal or a quick workout before an event. Staying active helps counterbalance occasional indulgences.

3. Practice Self-Awareness: Pay attention to your eating patterns and feelings during social events. If you find yourself eating out of habit or stress rather than hunger, take a moment to assess your needs.

4. Stay Hydrated: Drink plenty of water throughout the day and during social events. Sometimes thirst can be mistaken for hunger, leading to unnecessary snacking.

5. Use the 80/20 Rule: Follow the 80/20 rule, where you aim to make healthy choices 80% of the time and allow for some flexibility in the remaining 20%. This approach helps you

maintain a balanced perspective and prevents feelings of deprivation.

6. Seek Support: Share your goals with friends or family members who can offer support and encouragement. Having a support system can make it easier to stay on track.

By planning ahead for social events, making mindful choices at restaurants, and employing strategies to stay committed, you can enjoy social occasions without compromising your weight loss goals. The next chapter will focus on maintaining motivation and overcoming common obstacles on your weight loss journey.

PART IV:

LONG-TERM MAINTENANCE AND LIFESTYLE

10.

STAYING MOTIVATED

Successfully maintaining your weight loss and adopting a healthy lifestyle involves more than just following a diet—it's about integrating lasting habits and staying motivated over time. This section addresses key strategies for staying motivated, celebrating milestones, handling setbacks, and leveraging support systems.

Staying Motivated

1. Set Ongoing Goals:

- Continuously set new, achievable goals to keep yourself focused and motivated. These goals could be related to fitness, nutrition, or personal growth.

2. Track Your Progress:
   - Use journals, apps, or regular check-ins to monitor your progress. Seeing your achievements can boost motivation and reinforce positive behavior.

3. Find Enjoyable Activities:
   - Engage in physical activities and hobbies you enjoy. When you find pleasure in your routines, you're more likely to stick with them.

4. Visualize Success:
   - Regularly visualize your long-term goals and the benefits of maintaining a healthy lifestyle. Visualization helps keep your objectives clear and motivates you to continue.

5. Create a Routine:

- Develop a consistent routine that includes healthy eating and regular exercise. Routine helps integrate these behaviors into your daily life, making them feel like second nature.

Celebrating Small Wins

1. Acknowledge Milestones:
   - Celebrate each achievement, no matter how small. Recognizing your progress reinforces positive behavior and keeps you motivated.

2. Reward Yourself:
   - Choose non-food-related rewards for reaching your goals, such as a new outfit, a relaxing massage, or a fun outing. This helps create positive associations with your efforts.

3. Share Your Success:
   - Share your milestones with friends, family, or a support group. Celebrating with others can amplify your sense of accomplishment and encouragement.

4. Reflect on Progress:
   - Take time to reflect on how far you've come.
Reviewing your journey and the positive
changes you've made can boost your confidence
and motivation.

5. Document Achievements:
   - Keep a visual record of your successes, such
as before-and-after photos or progress charts.
This serves as a constant reminder of your hard
work and accomplishments.

Dealing with Setbacks

1. Stay Positive:
   - Maintain a positive mindset and view
setbacks as opportunities to learn and grow.
Acknowledge the challenge and refocus on your
goals.

2. Analyze the Situation:
   - Assess what led to the setback and identify
any patterns or triggers. Understanding these

factors can help you develop strategies to prevent future issues.

3. Adjust Your Plan:
   - Make necessary adjustments to your diet or exercise plan based on the insights gained from the setback. Flexibility is key to long-term success.

4. Seek Support:
   - Reach out to your support network or a professional for guidance and encouragement. Sometimes, external perspectives can offer valuable insights and motivation.

5. Practice Self-Compassion:
   - Be kind to yourself and avoid self-criticism. Understand that setbacks are a natural part of the journey and do not define your overall progress.

The Power of a Support System

1. Build a Network:

- Surround yourself with supportive friends, family, or a community group that shares your health and wellness goals. A strong network can offer encouragement and accountability.

2. Join Support Groups:
   - Participate in online or in-person support groups where you can share experiences, seek advice, and gain motivation from others facing similar challenges.

3. Engage with a Coach or Mentor:
   - Work with a health coach, dietitian, or mentor who can provide personalized advice, motivation, and support throughout your journey.

4. Communicate Openly:
   - Share your goals, challenges, and successes with your support network. Open communication fosters understanding and strengthens relationships.

5. Provide Support to Others:

- Offer support and encouragement to others on their own health journeys. Being a source of support not only benefits them but also reinforces your own commitment to a healthy lifestyle.

Maintaining long-term weight loss and a healthy lifestyle requires ongoing motivation, celebration of progress, resilience in the face of setbacks, and the strength of a supportive network. By focusing on these aspects, you can sustain your achievements and continue to thrive in your wellness journey.

11.

ADAPTING TO LIFE CHANGES

Life is full of transitions and major events that can impact your weight loss journey. Adapting your plan to fit different life stages and circumstances is essential for maintaining progress and well-being. This chapter will explore how to adjust your plan for various life stages, manage weight during pregnancy and menopause, and cope with major life events.

Adjusting Your Plan for Different Life Stages

As you move through different stages of life, your health needs and routines may change. Adapting your weight loss and wellness plan to fit these changes can help you stay on track.

1. Young Adulthood: In this stage, you may be dealing with new responsibilities, such as starting a career or managing a busy social life. Focus on establishing healthy habits and finding a balanced approach to eating and exercise that fits your schedule.

2. Midlife: During midlife, you might face changes in metabolism, activity levels, and family dynamics. Adjust your plan by incorporating regular physical activity, focusing on nutrient-dense foods, and addressing any emerging health issues.

3. Older Adults: As you age, muscle mass and metabolism can decrease. Emphasize strength training to maintain muscle mass, adjust calorie intake to reflect changes in metabolism, and ensure your diet includes adequate nutrients to support overall health.

Managing Weight During Pregnancy and Menopause

Pregnancy

Maintaining a healthy weight during pregnancy is important for both maternal and fetal health. Here are some guidelines for managing weight during this time:

1. Focus on Nutrient-Dense Foods: Emphasize a balanced diet rich in fruits, vegetables, whole grains, lean proteins, and healthy fats to support your baby's development and your own health.

2. Monitor Weight Gain: Follow your healthcare provider's recommendations for weight gain during pregnancy. Weight gain is a normal part of pregnancy, but it's important to monitor it to ensure it remains within healthy limits.

3. Stay Active: Engage in regular, moderate physical activity, such as walking or prenatal yoga, unless contraindicated by your healthcare provider. Exercise can help manage weight, improve mood, and support overall health.

4. Consult Your Healthcare Provider: Work closely with your healthcare provider to address any concerns about weight gain, nutrition, or exercise during pregnancy.

Menopause

Menopause can lead to changes in metabolism and hormone levels, affecting weight and body composition. Consider the following strategies:

1. Adjust Caloric Intake: As metabolism slows, you may need to adjust your caloric intake to prevent weight gain. Focus on nutrient-dense foods that provide essential vitamins and minerals.

2. Incorporate Strength Training: Strength training is important for maintaining muscle mass and bone density during menopause. Include exercises that build strength and support bone health.

3. Manage Symptoms: Address symptoms of menopause, such as hot flashes and mood swings, through lifestyle changes, stress management, and consulting your healthcare provider for appropriate treatments.

4. Focus on Hydration: Staying hydrated is important for overall health and can help manage symptoms such as bloating and weight fluctuations.

Coping with Major Life Events

Major life events, such as job changes, relocation, or the loss of a loved one, can impact your emotional well-being and disrupt your routines. Here's how to cope with these challenges:

1. Acknowledge Emotions: Recognize that major life events can affect your emotional state and eating habits. Allow yourself to feel and process these emotions without turning to food for comfort.

2. Maintain Routine: Try to maintain your healthy eating and exercise routines as much as possible, even during stressful times. Routine can provide stability and help you stay on track.

3. Seek Support: Reach out to friends, family, or a support group for emotional support and encouragement. Having a support network can help you navigate challenging times and stay focused on your goals.

4. Be Flexible: Understand that life changes may require adjustments to your plan. Be flexible and adapt your goals and strategies as needed to fit your current circumstances.

5. Prioritize Self-Care: Take time for self-care activities that promote relaxation and well-being, such as exercise, meditation, or hobbies. Self-care can help you manage stress and maintain a positive outlook.

By adjusting your plan to accommodate different life stages, managing weight during pregnancy and menopause, and coping with major life events, you can maintain your progress and overall health. The next chapter will focus on maintaining long-term success and continuing your journey towards a healthier lifestyle.

12.

MAINTAINING YOUR PROGRESS

Maintaining progress after achieving your weight loss goals is essential for long-term success and overall health. This chapter will discuss long-term strategies for success, the role of regular check-ins, and the importance of continuing to set and achieve goals.

Long-Term Strategies for Success

Sustaining your progress requires ongoing effort and commitment. Implementing these long-term strategies can help you stay on track and maintain a healthy lifestyle:

1. Adopt a Balanced Approach: Focus on a balanced diet and regular exercise as part of your daily routine rather than viewing them as

short-term fixes. This approach fosters lasting changes and helps prevent weight regain.

2. Stay Consistent: Consistency is key to maintaining progress. Establish routines that incorporate healthy eating, regular physical activity, and self-care. Make these habits a natural part of your lifestyle.

3. Monitor Your Progress: Keep track of your weight, fitness levels, and overall health through regular self-assessments. Monitoring your progress helps you stay accountable and identify any areas that may need adjustment.

4. Practice Mindful Eating: Continue to practice mindful eating by paying attention to hunger and fullness cues, enjoying your food, and making conscious food choices. This helps you maintain a healthy relationship with food.

5. Stay Educated: Keep learning about nutrition, exercise, and wellness. Staying informed can

help you make better choices and adapt to changes in your health or lifestyle.

The Role of Regular Check-Ins

Regular check-ins are vital for assessing your progress and making necessary adjustments to your plan. Consider these methods for effective check-ins:

1. Schedule Regular Assessments: Set specific times for self-assessments, such as monthly or quarterly, to review your weight, fitness levels, and overall health. This helps you track your progress and identify trends.

2. Evaluate Your Goals: Periodically review your goals and adjust them as needed. Celebrate your achievements and set new goals to keep yourself motivated and engaged.

3. Track Your Habits: Keep a journal or use an app to track your eating habits, exercise routines, and any changes in your weight or health. This

can provide valuable insights and help you stay on track.

4. Seek Professional Support: Consider working with a registered dietitian, personal trainer, or healthcare provider for periodic check-ins and guidance. They can offer personalized advice and support.

Continuing to Set and Achieve Goals

Setting and achieving new goals helps you stay motivated and focused on your long-term success. Here's how to continue setting and reaching your goals:

1. Set SMART Goals: Use the SMART criteria—Specific, Measurable, Achievable, Relevant, and Time-bound—when setting new goals. This approach ensures your goals are clear and attainable.

2. Break Goals into Smaller Steps: Divide larger goals into smaller, manageable steps. This makes

the goals less overwhelming and allows you to track progress more easily.

3. Stay Flexible: Be open to adjusting your goals as needed based on your progress and any changes in your life. Flexibility helps you adapt to challenges and stay on track.

4. Celebrate Milestones: Recognize and celebrate your achievements along the way. Celebrating milestones boosts motivation and reinforces positive behaviors.

5. Maintain a Positive Mindset: Keep a positive and resilient mindset, even when faced with setbacks or challenges. Focus on your progress and remind yourself of the reasons behind your goals.

6. Seek Support: Share your goals with friends, family, or a support group. Having a support system can provide encouragement and accountability.

By implementing long-term strategies for success, utilizing regular check-ins, and continuing to set and achieve goals, you can maintain your progress and enjoy a healthier lifestyle. The journey towards a healthier you is ongoing, and with commitment and perseverance, you can achieve lasting success.

PART V:

RECIPES AND MEAL IDEAS

13.

BREAKFAST IDEAS

Breakfast is an important meal that sets the tone for the rest of the day. Choosing nutritious options can help you stay energized and focused. This section offers quick and nutritious breakfast ideas, as well as high-protein recipes to support your weight loss goals and overall health.

Quick and Nutritious Options

1. Overnight Oats:
   - Ingredients: Rolled oats, chia seeds, almond milk, Greek yogurt, fresh fruit, honey.
   - Instructions: Combine oats, chia seeds, and almond milk in a jar. Stir and let sit overnight. In

the morning, add Greek yogurt, fresh fruit, and a drizzle of honey.

2. Avocado Toast:
  - Ingredients: Whole-grain bread, ripe avocado, cherry tomatoes, red pepper flakes, olive oil.
  - Instructions: Toast the bread and mash the avocado. Spread the avocado on the toast, top with sliced cherry tomatoes, and sprinkle with red pepper flakes and a drizzle of olive oil.

3. Smoothie Bowl:
  - Ingredients: Spinach, banana, frozen berries, Greek yogurt, almond milk, granola.
  - Instructions: Blend spinach, banana, frozen berries, Greek yogurt, and almond milk until smooth. Pour into a bowl and top with granola and additional fruit.

4. Greek Yogurt Parfait:
  - Ingredients: Greek yogurt, mixed berries, granola, honey.

- Instructions: Layer Greek yogurt with mixed berries and granola in a bowl or glass. Drizzle with honey.

5. Egg Muffins:
  - Ingredients: Eggs, spinach, bell peppers, onions, salt, pepper.
  - Instructions: Whisk eggs and season with salt and pepper. Stir in chopped spinach, bell peppers, and onions. Pour into muffin tins and bake at 375°F (190°C) for 20 minutes, or until set.

High-Protein Recipes

1. Veggie and Egg Scramble:
  - Ingredients: Eggs, spinach, mushrooms, bell peppers, onion, salt, pepper.
  - Instructions: Sauté vegetables in a pan until tender. Add beaten eggs and cook until scrambled and cooked through. Season with salt and pepper.

2. Protein-Packed Smoothie:

- Ingredients: Protein powder, banana, almond milk, spinach, chia seeds.
   - Instructions: Blend protein powder, banana, almond milk, spinach, and chia seeds until smooth. Enjoy as a high-protein, nutrient-rich breakfast.

3. Quinoa Breakfast Bowl:
   - Ingredients: Cooked quinoa, berries, Greek yogurt, almonds, honey.
   - Instructions: Top cooked quinoa with Greek yogurt, fresh berries, sliced almonds, and a drizzle of honey.

4. Turkey and Veggie Breakfast Wrap:
   - Ingredients: Whole-grain tortilla, sliced turkey breast, scrambled eggs, spinach, tomato.
   - Instructions: Place sliced turkey breast, scrambled eggs, spinach, and tomato on a tortilla. Roll up and enjoy.

5. Chia Seed Pudding:
   - Ingredients: Chia seeds, almond milk, vanilla extract, fresh fruit.

- Instructions: Mix chia seeds with almond milk and vanilla extract. Refrigerate for several hours or overnight until thickened. Top with fresh fruit before serving.

These breakfast ideas offer a variety of options to suit different tastes and dietary preferences, helping you start your day with energy and nutrition.

14.

LUNCH AND DINNER RECIPES

Creating balanced, nutritious meals for lunch and dinner is key to maintaining energy levels and supporting your weight loss goals. This section provides recipes for balanced meals that offer sustained energy, as well as plant-based and low-carb options to suit various dietary preferences.

Balanced Meals for Sustained Energy

1. Grilled Chicken Salad:
   - Ingredients: Grilled chicken breast, mixed greens, cherry tomatoes, cucumber, red onion, avocado, balsamic vinaigrette.
   - Instructions: Toss mixed greens with sliced cherry tomatoes, cucumber, red onion, and

avocado. Top with sliced grilled chicken and drizzle with balsamic vinaigrette.

2. Quinoa and Black Bean Stuffed Bell Peppers:
   - Ingredients: Bell peppers, cooked quinoa, black beans, corn, diced tomatoes, shredded cheese, cumin, chili powder.
   - Instructions: Preheat oven to 375°F (190°C). Mix quinoa, black beans, corn, diced tomatoes, and spices. Stuff bell peppers with the mixture, top with shredded cheese, and bake for 25-30 minutes until peppers are tender.

3. Salmon with Sweet Potato and Asparagus:
   - Ingredients: Salmon fillets, sweet potatoes, asparagus, olive oil, lemon juice, garlic powder, salt, pepper.
   - Instructions: Preheat oven to 400°F (200°C). Toss sweet potato cubes and asparagus with olive oil, salt, pepper, and garlic powder. Place salmon fillets on a baking sheet, drizzle with lemon juice, and bake for 15-20 minutes, along with the vegetables.

4. Turkey and Vegetable Stir-Fry:
   - Ingredients: Ground turkey, bell peppers, broccoli, snap peas, carrots, soy sauce, garlic, ginger, olive oil.
   - Instructions: Heat olive oil in a pan and cook ground turkey until browned. Add chopped vegetables and stir-fry with garlic and ginger. Add soy sauce and cook until vegetables are tender.

5. Lentil and Spinach Soup:
   - Ingredients: Green or brown lentils, spinach, diced tomatoes, carrots, celery, onion, vegetable broth, garlic, thyme.
   - Instructions: Sauté onion, garlic, carrots, and celery in a pot. Add lentils, diced tomatoes, vegetable broth, and thyme. Simmer until lentils are tender. Stir in spinach before serving.

Plant-Based and Low-Carb Options

Plant-Based Options

1. Chickpea and Spinach Curry:

- Ingredients: Chickpeas, spinach, diced
tomatoes, onion, garlic, ginger, curry powder,
coconut milk.
- Instructions: Sauté onion, garlic, and ginger
until fragrant. Add curry powder and cook for 1
minute. Stir in diced tomatoes and coconut milk.
Add chickpeas and simmer for 10 minutes. Stir
in spinach before serving.

2. Stuffed Sweet Potatoes:
- Ingredients: Sweet potatoes, black beans,
corn, avocado, salsa, cilantro.
- Instructions: Bake sweet potatoes at 400°F
(200°C) until tender. Split open and top with
black beans, corn, avocado slices, salsa, and
chopped cilantro.

3. Tofu and Vegetable Stir-Fry:
- Ingredients: Firm tofu, bell peppers, broccoli,
snow peas, soy sauce, sesame oil, garlic.
- Instructions: Press tofu to remove excess
moisture and cut into cubes. Sauté tofu until
golden. Add vegetables and stir-fry with garlic

and soy sauce. Finish with a splash of sesame
oil.

4. Vegetable and Hummus Wrap:
   - Ingredients: Whole-grain wrap, hummus,
cucumber, bell peppers, carrots, spinach.
   - Instructions: Spread hummus on the wrap
and layer with sliced vegetables and spinach.
Roll up tightly and slice in half.

5. Cauliflower Rice Bowl:
   - Ingredients: Cauliflower rice, black beans,
corn, diced tomatoes, avocado, lime juice.
   - Instructions: Sauté cauliflower rice until
tender. Top with black beans, corn, diced
tomatoes, and avocado slices. Drizzle with lime
juice.

Low-Carb Options

1. Zucchini Noodles with Pesto:
   - Ingredients: Zucchini, basil pesto, cherry
tomatoes, Parmesan cheese.

- Instructions: Spiralize zucchini into noodles and sauté briefly. Toss with basil pesto and cherry tomatoes. Top with grated Parmesan cheese.

2. Chicken Lettuce Wraps:
   - Ingredients: Ground chicken, bell peppers, onions, garlic, soy sauce, lettuce leaves.
   - Instructions: Cook ground chicken with chopped bell peppers, onions, and garlic. Season with soy sauce. Serve in lettuce leaves as wraps.

3. Eggplant Lasagna:
   - Ingredients: Eggplant slices, marinara sauce, ricotta cheese, mozzarella cheese, Parmesan cheese.
   - Instructions: Layer eggplant slices with marinara sauce and cheeses in a baking dish. Bake at 375°F (190°C) for 30-35 minutes.

4. Salmon and Avocado Salad:
   - Ingredients: Salmon fillets, mixed greens, avocado, cucumber, cherry tomatoes, lemon vinaigrette.

  - Instructions: Grill or bake salmon fillets and flake into pieces. Toss with mixed greens, sliced avocado, cucumber, and cherry tomatoes. Drizzle with lemon vinaigrette.

5. Stuffed Mushrooms:
  - Ingredients: Large mushroom caps, cream cheese, garlic, herbs, Parmesan cheese.
  - Instructions: Mix cream cheese with garlic and herbs. Stuff into mushroom caps and top with Parmesan cheese. Bake at 375°F (190°C) for 20 minutes.

These lunch and dinner recipes provide a variety of options to suit different dietary needs and preferences, helping you maintain balanced nutrition and energy throughout the day.

15.

SNACKS AND DESSERTS

Finding nutritious snacks and satisfying desserts is crucial for maintaining energy levels and curbing cravings while adhering to a healthy eating plan. This section provides ideas for healthy snacks and guilt-free desserts that support your weight loss goals and overall well-being.

Healthy Snack Ideas

1. Greek Yogurt with Berries:
   - Ingredients: Greek yogurt, fresh or frozen berries, honey (optional).
   - Instructions: Top a serving of Greek yogurt with berries. Drizzle with a little honey if desired.

2. Veggie Sticks with Hummus:

- Ingredients: Carrot sticks, celery sticks, bell pepper strips, hummus.

   - Instructions: Serve a variety of raw vegetable sticks with a portion of hummus for dipping.

3. Apple Slices with Almond Butter:
   - Ingredients: Apple, almond butter.
   - Instructions: Slice an apple and spread almond butter on each slice or serve as a dip.

4. Nuts and Seeds Mix:
   - Ingredients: Almonds, walnuts, sunflower seeds, pumpkin seeds.
   - Instructions: Combine a small handful of mixed nuts and seeds for a crunchy, nutrient-rich snack.

5. Cottage Cheese with Pineapple:
   - Ingredients: Cottage cheese, pineapple chunks (fresh or canned in juice).
   - Instructions: Mix cottage cheese with pineapple chunks for a sweet and satisfying snack.

6. Hard-Boiled Eggs:
   - Ingredients: Eggs.
   - Instructions: Boil eggs, peel, and enjoy with a sprinkle of salt and pepper.

7. Edamame:
   - Ingredients: Frozen edamame, salt.
   - Instructions: Cook edamame according to package instructions, season with a pinch of salt, and serve warm or chilled.

Guilt-Free Desserts

1. Chia Seed Pudding:
   - Ingredients: Chia seeds, almond milk, vanilla extract, fresh fruit.
   - Instructions: Mix chia seeds with almond milk and vanilla extract. Refrigerate until thickened. Top with fresh fruit before serving.

2. Baked Apples with Cinnamon:
   - Ingredients: Apples, cinnamon, a touch of honey or maple syrup (optional).

- Instructions: Core apples and sprinkle with cinnamon. Bake at 350°F (175°C) for 20-25 minutes until tender.

3. Frozen Banana Bites:
   - Ingredients: Bananas, dark chocolate (70% cocoa or higher), coconut flakes (optional).
   - Instructions: Slice bananas and dip in melted dark chocolate. Place on a parchment-lined tray and freeze. Sprinkle with coconut flakes if desired.

4. Berry Sorbet:
   - Ingredients: Mixed berries (fresh or frozen), a splash of lemon juice, a touch of honey or stevia (optional).
   - Instructions: Blend berries with lemon juice and sweetener if using until smooth. Freeze until firm, then scoop and serve.

5. Greek Yogurt Popsicles:
   - Ingredients: Greek yogurt, fruit puree (e.g., strawberry or mango), a touch of honey (optional).

- Instructions: Mix Greek yogurt with fruit puree and sweetener if desired. Pour into popsicle molds and freeze until solid.

6. Avocado Chocolate Mousse:
   - Ingredients: Ripe avocados, cocoa powder, honey or maple syrup, vanilla extract.
   - Instructions: Blend avocados with cocoa powder, sweetener, and vanilla extract until smooth and creamy. Chill before serving.

7. Almond Flour Cookies:
   - Ingredients: Almond flour, almond butter, egg, honey, baking soda.
   - Instructions: Mix almond flour with almond butter, egg, honey, and baking soda. Scoop onto a baking sheet and bake at 350°F (175°C) for 10-12 minutes.

These snack and dessert options provide healthy alternatives to traditional choices, helping you enjoy satisfying treats while staying aligned with your wellness goals.

CONCLUSION

16.

LOOKING FORWARD: A LIFELONG JOURNEY

Embarking on a journey toward weight loss and overall wellness is not just about reaching a specific goal; it's about embracing a lifelong commitment to a healthy lifestyle. As you continue this journey, consider the following aspects to sustain your progress and inspire others.

Embracing a Healthy Lifestyle

1. Cultivate Consistent Habits:
   - Adopt and maintain healthy eating and exercise habits as part of your daily routine. Consistency is key to long-term success and well-being.

2. Celebrate Your Achievements:
  - Acknowledge and celebrate your milestones and successes, no matter how small. Recognizing your achievements reinforces positive behavior and motivation.

3. Adapt and Evolve:
  - Understand that your needs and circumstances may change over time. Be flexible and willing to adapt your strategies to fit new goals, life stages, or challenges.

4. Prioritize Wellness:
  - Focus on overall well-being, including physical, mental, and emotional health. Balance is essential for a sustainable and fulfilling lifestyle.

5. Set New Goals:
  - Continuously set and pursue new goals to keep yourself motivated and engaged. Goals provide direction and a sense of purpose in your journey.

Staying Informed and Educated

1. Stay Current with Research:
   - Keep up with the latest research and developments in nutrition, fitness, and wellness. Being informed helps you make better decisions and adjust your approach as needed.

2. Seek Professional Advice:
   - Consult with healthcare professionals, dietitians, or fitness experts to receive personalized advice and support. Professional guidance can enhance your understanding and results.

3. Read and Learn:
   - Explore books, articles, and reputable sources of information related to health and wellness. Education empowers you to make informed choices and stay motivated.

4. Embrace Lifelong Learning:
   - Treat your health journey as an ongoing learning process. Stay curious and open to new

information and techniques that can benefit your well-being.

Encouraging Others on Their Journey

1. Share Your Experience:
   - Share your successes, challenges, and strategies with others who may be on a similar journey. Your experience can provide valuable insights and motivation.

2. Be a Source of Support:
   - Offer encouragement and support to friends, family, or colleagues who are working towards their own health goals. Positive reinforcement and empathy can make a significant difference.

3. Promote Healthy Living:
   - Advocate for and model healthy lifestyle choices. Leading by example can inspire others to adopt similar habits and make positive changes in their lives.

4. Celebrate Others' Successes:

  - Acknowledge and celebrate the achievements of those around you. Recognizing others' successes fosters a supportive and motivating environment.

5. Create a Community:
  - Engage in or create a community or support group focused on health and wellness. Being part of a group can provide additional motivation, accountability, and shared resources.

Embracing a healthy lifestyle is a lifelong journey filled with opportunities for growth and self-discovery. By staying informed, adapting to changes, and supporting others, you can continue to thrive and inspire those around you. Your commitment to wellness not only benefits you but also contributes to a broader movement towards healthier living.